Morgellons Disease

The Silent Pandemic

Armando Hernandez

*A self-funded finding and study of a major silent pandemic
attacking humans, pets, animals, and insects*

NEWMAN SPRINGS PUBLISHING
320 Broad Street
Red Bank, NJ 07701

First originally published by Newman Springs Publishing 2020

ISBN 978-1-64801-024-8 (Paperback)
ISBN 978-1-64801-025-5 (Digital)

Printed in the United States of America

Abstract

Morgellons disease is a highly contagious fungi. It can be transmitted by air; contact with the infected area; and contact with infected persons, pets, farm animals, wildlife, or insect. This has been undiagnosed or misdiagnose as shingle, Lyme disease, fibromyalgia, herpes, eczema, plaque psoriasis, AIDS, or cold sores.

Author's Views and Finding about Morgellons Disease

Morgellons disease is caused by a fungus named *Aspergillus fumigatus*. This fungus is highly contagious and anyone can be infected by contact with an infected area, pet, and person, including sexual contact. The information about *Aspergillus fumigatus* in the Centers for Disease Control and Prevention (CDC), a government site, is not even close to how bad these fungi really are and what part the body it is attacking.

Morgellons disease (*Aspergillus fumigatus*) does not discriminate if you're young, old, rich, poor, black, or white. Once infected, the disease will spread rapidly. It is a worldwide pandemic and highly contagious. Most people are in denial until the fungus grows big enough to start interfering with your well-being. The biggest problem we have is that this organism has been spreading unimpeded on a worldwide scale. Believe it or not, this is a very scary situation. Through my research, I have seen what this organism is capable of doing. Some of the things you will see and feel will test your sanity.

Morgellons disease is a highly aggressive organism that is always looking to spread.

Dermatologists have been doing an injustice to their patients by diagnosing them as having delusions of parasitosis (DOP). This is why many people have attempted to take their lives because the doctors are telling their patients that they are crazy, and people have nowhere to go for help. DOP is in the government's National Library of Medicine (NLM) as the diagnosis for Morgellons disease when they are not referring to shingles, Lyme disease, fibromyalgia, eczema, dermatitis, cold sores, and herpes—all of which are Morgellons disease, which is caused by the fungus, *Aspergillus fumigatus.*

In the past ten years, this scary fungus has become the most common and life-threatening opportunistic fungal pathogen of the world. Part of the reasons is because it's living in plain sight. It's in front of you. You better wake up because this fungus is not just attacking people, animals, and insects, these fungi are destroying everything that lives.

One of the scariest thoughts that I had when I found out about these fungi was why the bees are starting to disappear. This may be one of the reasons why I've seen these fungi in action, attacking the insect population. It is not a pretty sight.

How I Got Infected with
Morgellons Disease

In 1999, I came in contact with some person at my computer and network store. At that time, I saw something for a fraction of a second that rendered me in a state of shock. I could not believe it so I convince myself that what I saw was just my imagination. It was so unbelievable that I felt that it was better for me to deny what I saw.

A few of days later, I started getting rashes throughout my body so I went to the doctors to have it checked out. They gave me some cream. This went on for a long time. I kept going back to the doctors with this very itchy problem, especially under the armpits and crotch area. The doctors diagnosed me with multiple problems: dermatophytosis, seborrheic dermatitis, xerotic eczema, ringworm, and scabies.

The situation went on for years. I started gaining weight and losing mobility as my arthritis got worse and worse. Even though I'm a very resourceful individual, I ended up losing my business as a computer and network consultant due to illness, loss of mobility, and pain.

By 2012, I started feeling massive amount of pain that came out of nowhere. The next year, I was practically bedridden. Finding ways to keep my house and feed my family was not easy after I lost the ability to work. Every time I went to the doctors, they can't figure out why I was what was causing all the pain. My regular doctor was very understanding. We worked together, compared our finding, and kept trying to understand what was medically wrong with me. Unfortunately, because the way the medical system is set up, he had no choice but to refer me to a so-called specialist. This is where we lost traction.

I had moments when my leg would swell up. The doctors would try to figure out if I had gout. I had moments when my leg would suddenly erupt in pain, like an electrical shock, and felt like my leg was breaking in half. Doctors thought I may have neuropathy but could never give me a solid answer. As time went on, the symptoms were getting worst. I was desperate as the itching and pain started to become unbearable.

In 2013, I started feeling things like crawling all over my body and face. The doctors kept saying I was imagining things that were not there. I went to a dermatologist who told me I was delusional, even though there were ugly looking red only skin. They kept trying to refer me to mental health. I also went to the eye doctors because my vision was getting worst. I also believe that there was something in there, but the eye doctor kept saying there is nothing there, and that the reason for my sight going bad is because of my age. From 2013 to 2014, I started investing a lot of money that I did not have and spent a lot time on the web looking for answers and experimenting on my own. Along with a lot of the treatments, the doctors also advised me to wash with benzoyl peroxide that did nothing for me other than dry my skin, which made it hard for me to sleep.

I bought a bottle of Nutrasilver colloidal silver to my doctor's appointment. I had already taken the dosage that morning, which made me feel better, but was advised by the doctor not to take because it would turn me blue. I asked the doctor, "Okay, what do you have for me that would help me?| The doctor then said, "Nothing, other than you are delusional. What you're feeling is not real (even though there were sores everywhere on my body)." I said to the doctor, "Do you think I gave a damn if I turn pink with polka dots! If you have nothing to give me and this thing helps me and makes me feel a little better, I am going to take it!"

That was the last time I went to the doctors for help. I was better off alone. It did not matter what evidence and lab work I brought to the doctors. They would look at me like I had two heads and practically ignore everything I said. We, the patients, are like sheep being led to slaughter. I had found so many people being told the same thing worldwide.

What Is Morgellons Disease?

In June 2014, I started looking for answers on my own because I knew I was not going to get help from doctors. From all the hell I was going through, I had to help myself or I would suffer a lot more than I already had. I would have gone crazy or die. During the first half of the year, I started looking for answers throughout the Web to find what people like myself were going through and how doctors were treating them like nut jobs.

I was convinced that an amoeba, insect, fungi, or something like that was living inside me. During this time, I try just about anything. As a precaution, please do not try these things:

- I poured pure bleach on my head in the shower so the fungus would turn to mucus thoughout my whole body. I thought I was going to choke to death, which went on for about thirty minutes. A few hours later, I rushed to the emergency room at around two in the morning because I felt this huge mass of something moving up my back toward the top of my head. It scared the hell out of me. However, I got no help from the medical field. They still thought I was crazy.
- Another time, I thought I poured some kind of acid on my head that turned the fungus to white puss. It looked like goo on the side of my face near the eyes, which scared the hell out me. I only wish I thought of getting a camera and take a picture. This was not my first thought since I was scared people from the medical field would tell me I was crazy.

Again, *please* do not try these things!

The Blue Bucket and Red Cup of Truth

When I finally found the beginning of the end, this is when I started to put everything together. Around July 2014, I started bathing with water and vinegar. I had to keep my eyes closed since the vinegar would have hurt my eyes. I poured vinegar to a bucket full of water. I used a red cup to pour the vinegar solution over my head then scrubbed my body. There was a time when I felt something fighting to stay attached to my body. I wished that I could have open my eyes just to see what was going on.

This is a very scary moment to be infected with something you can't see but feel all over your body. While I was still going through all these problems, people I did not even know or have ever met contacted me from my postings on the Internet. These people was so scared. I can understand what they were going through. This is why I was posting a lot of the information on what I found online. It is very scary to believe in certain things that test your sanity, especially when you're being told by so-called experts that there is nothing there.

I left the blue bucket and the red cup in the shower. After a while, I went back to clean it up. I was shocked to find particles floating in the water. This is when I finally started to put some of what was going on together. To this day, I still did not know what exactly it was, but it was solid evidence that there was something. I brought specimens, the image below, and other images to my doctor and medical experts. My doctor was amazed and referred me to the dermatologists. They were still stuck to the idea that I was delusional.

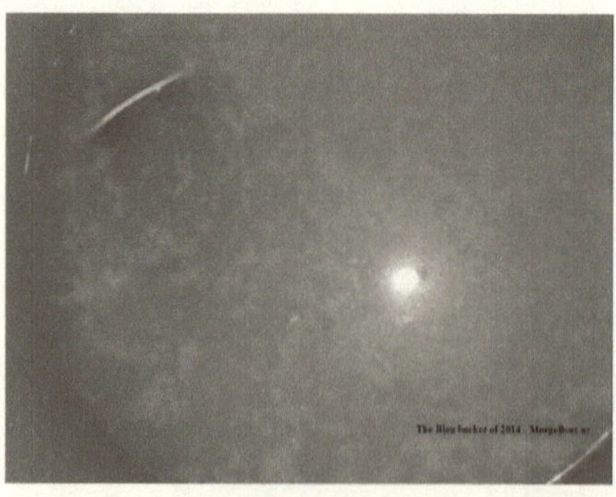

At this time, I am still trying to find some way to get this stuff off me, but every time I bathed with vinegar and water I would feel better for a short time. This went on for months. I was getting tired and feeling drained. Even though the doctors said I was not contagious, I knew they were wrong. I kept to myself all day in my home office and stayed away from everyone, including my family, for a long time.

I started investing a lot of money that I did not have, trying to find a cure. In October 2014, I put up my first video about my research on YouTube. In this first video, I was determined that my condition was caused by a fungus from everything I read, thought I did not have confirmation yet. I spent hundreds of hours contacting the CDC, local and national, but got nowhere. I had also contacted Center for Infectious Disease Research, but I also got nowhere with this. I invested hour trying to get samples to labs to be tested and kept getting denied. Even though I would pay cash or credit for it, they did not want to do it. I had to be a doctor or had a degree to submit samples for tests.

In December 2014, I made my second video about Morgellons disease and claimed it was an infestation by an amoeba or amoeba-like parasite (fungus), a living organism, but still no confirmation of any results at this time. In January 2015 I was convinced that Morgellons disease was caused by an infestation, but I still did not have the evidence of lab work since I was being block from submitting samples to labs. No matter how hard I try to get a doctor to submit the samples, they would still claim that I was crazy or delusional. It is very hard to restrain yourself from losing your temper with these doctors keep trying to send you to the physiatrist because you do not fall in line with the BS they are selling to us. What in the world happened to common sense!

In early spring of 2015, I found out that a medical group was having a conference in April at Austin, Texas. Even though I was financially strapped, I managed to sign up to see where they were on their research, if they had a cure or treatment, and if there was any way I could help. At the conference, the first thing one speaker said was that they already eliminated fungus as the cause of Morgellons disease. I was shocked to hear this because all my research brought me back to a fungus. Even though I was not an expert, I was certain they were wrong. I was able to talk to some speakers, I met one who had access to labs and asked if I could send some samples to him. He agreed. I got his business card with an address to send specimen. When I asked him about when we could make progress on finding the cause and cure, he said maybe ten years to find the cause. My mouth dropped, and I thought, Oh, hell no! There is no way in hell I could survive that long. This thing was driving me crazy with the brain fog, itch, and pain.

I met a lot of people who were suffering and looking desperately for help. I spoke with a few of them and found that they had been following my posts on YouTube, even though I never identified myself on my channel, Morgellonsus. Some of these people recognized my voice. They told me they follow my posting and agreed with what I was posting about Morgellons disease.

When I returned home, I immediately sent samples to the professor from the Austin convention. I waited for some response but got nothing from the professor. In August 2015, I found ways to get around labs not accepting my samples and specimen at a lab in the Boston area. I expected that the result would come back as fungus, but the microanalysis of the skin sample I sent (report number 831545) came back as a bacteria similar to *Alcaligenes faecalis*. I was devastated because I could not believe that it came back as bacteria when I knew that this was a fungus of fungi and this threw a curve on what I knew it was.

During this time, I started looking online and in the government medical library. I basically got my hopes up when an Israeli scientist found a fungus that have been masquerading as bacteria. In a way, I was happy from being somewhat vindicated. Despite my financial situation, I sent another multiple sample to the same company. Skin report number 1127151009 came back with a bacteria similar to *Clostridium innocuum*. According to the US National Library of Medicine, *Clostridium innocuum* is found in AIDS patients. In November 2015, I sent multiple samples to (FAL), and they came back with many different organisms: gram-positive cocci, *Kytococcus aerola-*

tus, and *Paenibacillus odorifer.* This was still not what I was looking for, but I was getting close. Financial burden was the main thing that was making it more complicated so I had to be selective on what I sent.

In January 2016, I sent more samples to FAL, and they came back with a fungus called *Penicillium citrinum,* known to be used to make penicillin. This was great. I finally started getting close to what I was looking for—the real source of the problem. In April 2016, I sent more samples to FAL. They came back with yeast. Again, I was getting even closer to the source of Morgellons disease. On April 12, 2016, I sent more samples to Sure-BioChem Laboratories, LLC. They came back with a fungus-mold *Penicillium chrysogenum.* On April 19, 2016, I sent more samples to FAL, and they came back with *Burkholderia pyrrocinia* or *Burkholderia cepacian, Staphylococcus epidermidis, Staphylococcus heamolyticus, Staphylococcus hominis,* or *Penicillium chrysogenum.* Again, I was getting even closer to the source of Morgellons disease. I invested a lot of time trying to find labs that does organism DNA and ID.

Austin Medical Conference on Morgellons Disease (April 2016)

I made sure that I got to the convention the day before because I was excited to help these people find the answers. The first thing I heard from these speakers during their beginning of introduction was that fungus was eliminated as the cause of Morgellons disease.

I ran into a lot of people that follow my YouTube channel. They were shocked to hear what these so-called experts telling us. I tried to give them what I had found and how I found it, but they would not accept anything other than their conclusion. As the first day ended, they kept congratulating themselves on how great everything went. I know this happened because other people brought it to my attention.

At the end of the first day function, I went to the hotel bar to enjoy a drink. Some people followed me there to speak with me and ask me how they could help themselves. It was not long after that a woman, who was either a physical therapist or psychiatrist, came to me, looking for help on how to get rid of this monster. I gave her some of the ideas that I had at that time. I also told her about Diflucan, which required a prescription. I asked the woman about her symptoms because she did not look like she had any visible sores or rash. She immediately pointed to the Band-Aid on her nose, which she covered with a lot of makeup.

As we spoke, a middle-aged woman came up to us and told us about some of the doctors who were helping her. They prescribed her to take certain drugs for about seven days. After that, they would give her different drugs. I told the woman that she should ask her doctors what they are treating her for. After all, how can they give her drugs to treat something if they don't know what they are treating. It is crazy when doctors say, "Let's just give them a drug. Yeah, that will cure it."

I went through the rest of the convention, realizing this was a waste of time. These people were in it for the glory, not concerned about the suffering that is going on worldwide right now.

In summer 2016, I got an appointment with a different doctor with a background in infectious disease and dermatology outside my normal network, trying to find someone who can identify the organism that invaded my body. I brought him a good specimen to analyze. He said my problem was a product of delusion and pointed to all the degrees on his wall, telling me that he has been doing this for many years and he knows what he was talking about. I, of course, told him that I believe he needed to go back to school. That was the final time that I try to give them help and guide them.

On November 9, 2016, I obtained an unbelievable specimen that was fully intact. I sent the samples to Sure-BioChem Laboratories, LLC for ID and DNA analysis. They came back with a fungus as *Aspergillus fumigatus*, the source of Morgellons disease. The lab used M192 DNA sequencing analysis for fungal isolates for result. When I got the results, I questioned the labs multiple times if there was any way the results could be wrong. They told me that there is no way, especially when they got hundred percent match to what is on file at the GenBank database at the National Center for Biotechnology Information's website. The DNA result confirms Aspergillus fumigatus as the main source of Morgellons disease and bacteria are secondary to the fungi. This fungus is able to hide in plain sight.

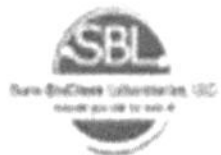

Sure-BioChem Laboratories, LLC

200 Federal Street, Suite 300, Camden, NJ 08103   (888) 398-7247

Client:	Hernandez		Order ID:	HERI 110916-01
			Date Received:	11/9/2016
	Shogun, MA		Date Analyzed:	11/9/2016
Attention:	Hernandez		Date Reported:	12/8/2016
Project:	Morgellons Epidemic		Date Amended:	

M192 DNA Sequencing Analysis for Fungal Isolates

Species Identification:

Species identity is based on the unknown organism's DNA sequence data for ITS region and the comparison to the GenBank database at the National Center for Biotechnology Information (www.ncbi.nlm.nih.gov). The PCR and DNA sequences were performed using universal fungal primers ITS4 and ITS5 DNA barcode primers. The DNA sequences were analyzed using BLAST search at NCBI.

Summary of Analysis

Lab Sample ID	Client Sample ID	Fungal Species Identified	Identity (%)
S6741-2	M 1	*Aspergillus fumigatus*	100%

```
CCCTCTGGGTCCAACCTCCCACCCGTGTCTATCGTACCTTGTTGCTTCGGCGGGCCCGCCGTTTCGACGGCCGCCGGGGAGGCCCTGCGCCCCCGGGC
CCGCGCCGCCGAAGACCCCAACATGAACGCTGTTCTGAAAGTATGCAGTCTGAGTTGATTATCGTAATCAGTTAAAACTTTCAACAACGGATCTCTT
GGTTCCGGCATCGATGAAGAACGCAGCGAAATGCGATAAGTAATGTGAATTGCAGAATTCAGTGAATCATCGAGTCTTTGAACGCACATTGCGCCCCC
TGGTATTCCGGGGGGCATGCCTGTCCGAGCGTCATTGCTGCCCTCAAGCACGGCTTGTGTGTTGGGCCCCCGTCCCCCTCTCCCGGGGGACGGGCCCG
AAAGGCAGCGGCCGCACCGCGTCCGGTCCTCGAGCGTATGGGGCTTTGTCACCTGCTCTGTAGGCCCGGCCGGCGCCAGCCGACACCCAACTTTATTT
TTCTAAGGTTGACCTCGGATCAGGTAGGGATACCCGCTGAACTTAAGCATATC
```

Zhencai Wu, M.S.
DNA Laboratory Manager

What Is Aspergillus Fumigatus?

According to NLM, Aspergillus fumigatus is an airborne fungus. While it was not the most dominant airborne fungus, over the past ten years, it has become the dominant airborne pathogen. I agree with what the national library, but it is not even close to how bad Aspergillus fumigatus is and how fast it is spreading worldwide.

It is highly contagious and can be transmitted by air, by contact (including sexual contact), and by residue left by a host. Aspergillus fumigatus does not discriminate against humans (male, female, black, or white), pets, farm animals, insects, or all wildlife. Once infected, you become the host. You do not even realize that you have a living organism growing on and inside your body. Inexplicably, you start gaining weight. Aspergillus fumigatus multiplies rapidly inside a host, spreading throughout the body like a thin blanket with multiple layers. Once a mycelium is created, the fungus begins the mass production. Like a nursery, the host will begin to produce spores that could spread in the air. The host will start feeling listless, weak and, depressed because the body is spending a lot of energy fighting off a fungal infection. There will be times when you feel like you got particles flying around you. These particles are spores. I was able to capture some and put them under the microscope. I saw what resembled colorful threads.

Aspergillus Fumigatus in a Specimen Jar

As I was getting specimen ready to send a sample to the labs, I found that one of the organisms was climbing the side of the specimen jar, so I pull out the microscope to take some image for the record. I was able get a picture of the fungus and the neural network it creates.

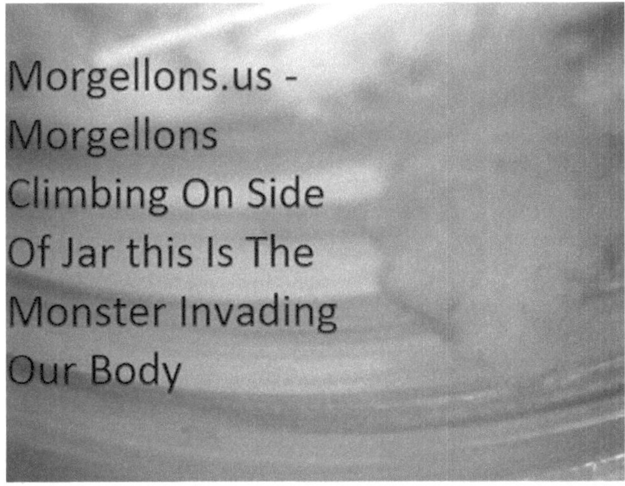

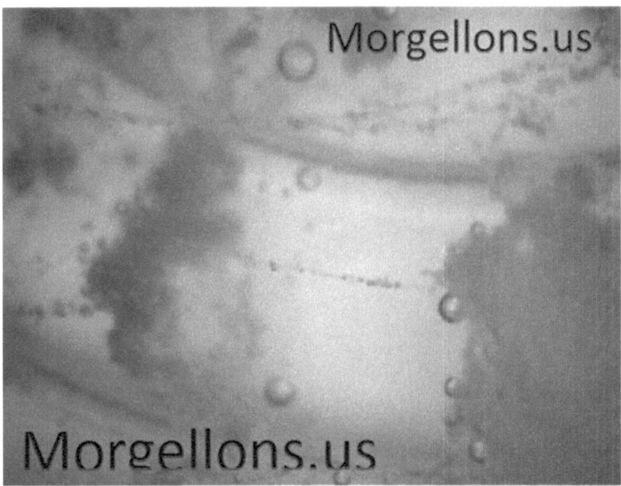

I had one sample in a specimen tube that I had left uncovered overnight. When I came back the next day, the specimen turn solid and apparently cracked the test tube. This blew my mind. I did not know what this was. I only knew that it was a living organism that is spreading worldwide unimpeded. I could not believe these fungi are able to morph, change shapes, turn to as hard as a rock, and turn to liquid. The medical field better get their head out of their behind before it is too late.

Now I Knew What I Was Fighting

Now that I knew what was fighting, I tried to show doctors to convince them that what I had was caused by a fungus. I gave them a copy of the DNA and other fungal reports that I got, but they still looked at me like I had two heads and that I was nuts. There are poor souls are out there who are weak, suffering, and going through the hell they are going through but are practically slapped in the face by the people who are supposed to help them.

I am a very resourceful individual so if the medical field would not give me what I needed to cure myself, even though I was financially broke, I would find a way to get it. I tried to find how to buy antifungal medicine to kill the fungus. At first, I was able to obtain Diflucan from Canada, but it was so expensive that I could not afford to continue buying it for very long. I was running out of money. It was very hard to be able to feed myself and family due to inability to maintain gainful work. Soon after, I found a way to get two kilos of fluconazole (Diflucan) from oversea. I started to make my own capsule of fluconazole and took it three times a day. Within a short time, I noticed the the fungus started shrinking. I knew that I was in process of killing the infestation. Originally, I really wanted to buy Vfend (voriconazole), but I could not buy it from Canada and it cost $9,000 per gram to get it from oversea. I could not afford that, which was how is I ended up with fluconazole. There are some natural products that are just as strong as fluconazole, but I did not know that at this time. However, I have passed the information on to the people that view my YouTube channel.

I was very excited that my life started getting better, I was starting to win the battle with Morgellons disease (*Aspergillus fumigatus*), and that the medical convention in Austin was a few days away so I could share my findings with the so-called expert scientists.

Austin Medical Conference on Morgellons Disease
(April 2017)

I was planning to go the medical conference on Morgellons disease in Austin, Texas, and already paid to attend. I planned to share with them all my data and reports that I had obtain from lab works I submitted. The people in charge of the medical conference disinvited me a few days later and sent back a refund. They told me that I was causing trouble and cornering people to speak with me. This was a total lie. They also suggested me that I should set up my own conference so I could share my data. So are these medical conferences really looking for the truth or fame and fortune?

I was willing to give information away as long they were going to help the people that were suffering, but now I was being force to do things I did not want to do. I decided that I was going to go public, but I ended up changing my decision. Instead, I was going to run for office, even though my family hate publicity. That was one of the problems I would have had with going public, but I spoke with family and got the okay from my spouse and family. So instead of flying to Texas for the medical conference, I ended up flying to Washington DC on the same weekend to take classes in Arlington, Virginia, about running for office. I went through the process but was not able to obtain enough signatures in time to get on the ballot. I was experiencing some chills and was not able to go out in cold weather.

Even though I was in process of the killing the fungus invading my body, I was still taking a beating from the only symptom I had left.

When Did Our Skin Become Transparent?

Morgellons patients claim about seeing that you have threads underneath their skin with microscope and are told by doctors and so-called experts that it is unexplained dermopathy and other claim psychosis called "DPO." The question I have—and everyone else should ask—are, when did your skin become transparent, how in the world can you see threads underneath your skin, and, on top of that, when did the skin resemble silicone? My god, these questions were so easy to answer. If your skin is not supposed to be transparent and looks like silicon, then why are we not looking to see why your skin is covered with a transparent silicon-like coat? When did half the human race become so stupid to be led like sheep to a slaughter?

The doctors throughout the world have to start using their head and troubleshoot. What they don't understand is that the world is in grave danger from an organism that is getting larger and larger every day that goes by and preys on every living thing. Don't they understand that these fungi are going after everybody and everything, including insects, livestock, wildlife, and pets? Doctors and scientists are either being led by either greed or stupidity. Neither of these is a good choice.

If we do not start working together to control or destroy this organism, the world and the human race is doomed. Babies can be infected from contact with an infected mother. We need to work together or the human race is in danger of extinction. This is a highly contagious living organism.

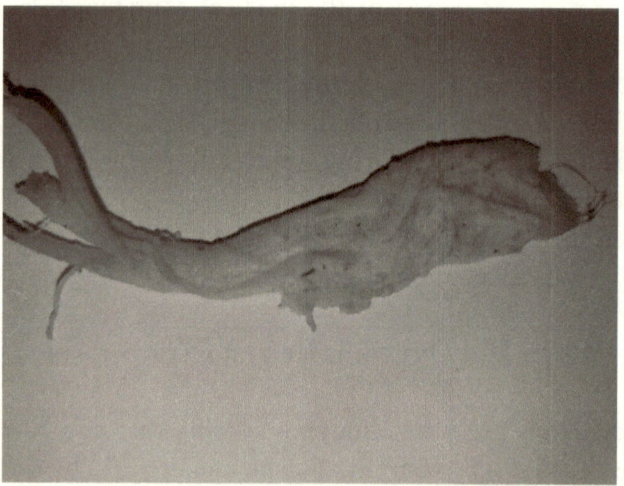

Some Conversations I Had with Other People Worldwide

In the summer of 2016, I started being contacted by many people, poor and rich, begging for me help. I have gotten e-mails from people who were ready to end their lives, devastated with their condition.

A woman from Tennessee e-mailed me and told me that she try to kill herself twice. She was happy that she found the data I was putting up on YouTube. I replied to her e-mail and asked for her phone number. As soon as she gave me her number, I called her back, like I do with all the people who asked me for help. I told her she can win this battle, that she's not alone, and that I would never quit to find the source of the disease because I was worried about my family and friends. She told me that she didn't want to die, but when she went to the doctors, they told her there was nothing there, that she's crazy, and that she needed to see psychiatrist, even though she knew it was real.

I have spoken with another family in Tennessee, a mother of two kids and her mother who has been suffering with Morgellons disease. She had to deal with her kids being ill and worried that her kids infecting other kids. On top of that, when the kids were too ill to go to school from the pain, she had take the kids to the doctors who would ust tell her there was nothing wrong with them. She called a few weeks later, screaming about something. At that time, I was concerned about her state of mind because what she was telling me something was coming out of the toilet to get to her. It sounded crazy.

Another couple from Michigan told me that they saw their carpet rise up. They were asking me how they could treat their home.

Now just to be clear, I'm not putting these people in the funny farm. I understand their experience and could believe they probably did experience something. I experienced a similar situation. The main sewer line got clogged in my house one time. Everything stated coming out of the first-floor shower drain, and the toilet would not flush. Since my home was about eight feet above street level, the drain was a straight shot, draining down toward the street, so it is very hard to clog. I climbed up on the roof and used a plumber snake down the main line. After I ran a hundred feet, I pulled it out, and it came back with strands of hair like fibers. But the line was still clogged so I poured vinegar in the toilet. Almost immediately, the drain opened up. Shortly after that, I told everyone to keep a gallon of white vinegar next to the toilet.

I spoke with another woman from Texas who sent me an e-mail, begging me to help her. She said she wanted to die because she can't stand the hell she was going through. I found her phone number on the Internet so I called her for two reasons—one, to ask if could delete her phone number and, the other, to try to help her. When I called her, the poor woman was crying right from the start, stuck in her room. She told me that she had no friends anymore or people who would help her. She could barely move from the pain, and the bites and itching were unbearable. I gave her some idea on what to do with what she may already have in her kitchen to treat herself. I also kept telling her that she will win this battle, don't give up, and just do what I told her then she will be okay. "You will win," I said.

I was on the phone with her for over an hour, trying to comfort her and telling she would be okay. This call really pulls on my heartstrings. I can't believe that the doctors would let someone suffer this much. About a week passed, I got a phone call from her. She was very excited. She told me she was at Walmart, asking me what about the other stuff I told her to buy. I was totally shocked. I asked, "Are you at Walmart? I thought you were bedridden?" She said that she had tried some of the things I told her, and she was getting better. She even worked in her garden that morning. Then she asked again about the other stuff I told her to buy. The feeling of getting a call like that from a person who was ready to end it all was amazing. I had to become a counselor to these people who are begging for help and scared to talk to medical professionals because they would claim the patients are nuts.

I spoke with another couple from Texas who went to see dermatologist. The doctor examined the sores as the patient explained that the sores won't heal. Somehow the patient mentioned Morgellons disease. Then the doctor told the patient, "You'll be okay. You have DOP (delusions of parasitosis)."

Another couple from Illinois recently contacted for help because a well-known dermatologist told the woman she had DOP and recommended her to a psychiatrist. I had spoken with other people who were locked up in the psych ward for going to doctors.

I had a very well off individual from California contact me, driven nuts by feeling something moving on his face. He was very angry with doctors who kept trying to tell him he was delusional.

I gave him a lot of information on what he could take and which doctor could give him a drug to treat and kill these fungi. He went to see his doctor to try to get him what he needed, but the doctor called him delusional again. He took his file and walk out of the office because got fed up with the deafness of these puppets.

Another couple from Southern California said that they would drive to Mexico to get the antifungal drug to treat the fungus. A veteran from Texas believes that he lost some limbs from Morgellons disease. I had giving him a lot of things he could try. I also suggested telling the doctors to treat for a fungus, not use the m-word (Morgellons disease), play stupid, and try to guide the doctor to the right road. He tried it and was able to get at least Diflucan, which will help, but it was not the one he wanted.

I have spoken with hundreds of people suffering worldwide. They all have been treated worse off or just as bad as the people I listed here. They all felt the same way about the medical field. This madness has to stop!

Eczema Commercials, Morgellons Disease, and the Medical Field

Eczema is spreading like wildfire throughout the world. Eczema commercials claim the same thing that Morgellons disease patients claim, yet Eczema patients are not called nuts or have DOP. The eczema commercials show antlike things crawling on the skin even though you cannot see it, like a snake slithering all over your body.

Come on, people! Start using your brain. We claim that we humans are the smartest life form in the globe, yet we accept the BS we are fed with. Morgellons disease is not a disease. It is infestation by a highly aggressive fungus called *Aspergillus fumigatus*.

How You Catch Morgellons Disease

Morgellons disease is spreading like wildfire throughout the world, spread by air, residue, and touch (includes sexual contact). Once you come in contact with the fungus, it grows very slow growth, but it keeps growing and growing. Fungi reproduce asexually, which means that it does not require more than one to reproduce. Once it is on you, it will immediately start reproducing and spread throughout your whole body, including the inside. It will look for the best place to anchor itself to you. The best location is on the head, under the hair.

Soon the fungus starts to grow and develop what is called a mycelium, which will be the nursery for mass production. As the fungus grows, your vision will start getting blurry. The happens because you are looking through multiple layers of glass (silicon). The fungus will be clear, just like it is throughout your whole body. As time goes on, the layers become thicker and thicker. You will start finding threads throughout your whole body, which is actually the hyphae come in from one of the mycelium. The growth will build a neural network connecting all the mycelium throughout your whole body.

From the moment you get infected, you experience a lot of itching. As time goes on, you start getting joint pains on your knees, ankles, feet, back, legs, shoulders, arms, elbows, wrist, hand, fingers, and your neck, which would get worse and worse. You will also start getting a hacking cough and runny nose. This is not a cold or a flu.

The process is very slow and complicated. At a certain time, you start realizing that you're having a problem that will only keep getting worst.

Morgellons Disease Symptoms

- *Eyes*
  - Blurry vision.
    - The reason why you get blurry vision is because you are looking through multiple layers of glass. Morgellons is covering your body, including your eyes, with multiple layers of silicon.
    - I went to the eye doctor to explain to him that I had something inside my eye that was sometimes very painful. I saw them multiple times, and they said they found nothing. Every time I visited the doctors, I kept telling them to wear gloves because

I knew I was contagious. They would look at me weirdly. I gave up on my doctors eventually because it did me no good to go there.

- Your eyes are the reason why it is so hard to treat and kill these fungi. I will explain on the treatment chapter and describe everything you need to do to help with your eyesight problem.

- *Head*
  - Your head will feel very lumpy. You will find sore like craters, some that are very painful in certain areas.
  - Sometimes you may notice that your head seems to look larger than it's supposed to be, like it's swelling up like a balloon. It is somewhat true, but it is not your head.
  - Your hair starts turning white and transparent, which it is not really hair.
  - You may grow a full white-gray beard, even though you could never grow a full beard before.

- *Headaches and Migraines*
  - You will get headaches and migraine. If your head ever felt it was solid and hard like a rock, it is not your head. It is the fungi turning solid and squeezing your head.

- *Concentration and Depression*
  - With brain fog, your ability to think and concentrate gets very complicated. You will find it a little hard to remember some things.
  - I think that Morgellons disease (*Aspergillus fumigatus*) may be what really causes Alzheimer's disease.
  - During the time I was looking for the cause of Morgellons disease, I found a lot of similar signs and symptoms of Alzheimer's. Something that led me to believe that *Aspergillus fumigatus* may be the real cause of Alzheimer's.
  - I will be looking further into Alzheimer's disease in the near future.

- ○ You will feel very depressed because you and your body is taking a beating, trying to fight off these invaders.
- ○ Inability to concentrate or focus.
- *Body*
  - ○ dry, rough, and scaly patches
  - ○ weight gain or weight loss
  - ○ blistering
  - ○ red rash
  - ○ chronic fatigue, weakness, and physically always tired
  - ○ lower back pain, neck pain, and shoulder pain
  - ○ change in appetite (increase or decrease)
  - ○ feet, knee, and hand swelling
  - ○ joint pain
  - ○ muscle cramping or twitching
  - ○ disorientation and dizziness
  - ○ arthritis throughout your whole body
  - ○ bloating
  - ○ blood pressure problems (low or high)
  - ○ severe itching
  - ○ fever or chills
  - ○ lower back pain
  - ○ stools looks different and may contain foreign looking matter
  - ○ painful skin cracking
  - ○ stomach bloating, looks and feels like it is moving
  - ○ pain coming out of nowhere
  - ○ numb sensation on body parts
  - ○ lesions appear out of nowhere and may disappear within a few minutes or longer
  - ○ ingrown hair that is hard to remove and extremely painful
  - ○ hair strands that are unusually thick and doesn't look like the other hair
  - ○ fingernails change shape and/or texture; becomes very brittle, crack, and break easily

- o fiber or threadlike material breaking from the skin or visible just beneath the skin, which may be red, blue, black, white, or clear
- o some fibers may move
- o lumps throughout your whole body
- o painful sore in your leg or other parts of your body
- *Nose, Sinus, and Throat*
    - o runny nose with constant mucus
    - o scratchy throat
    - o sneezing (you may sneeze out a ball of fibers)
    - o sneezing attack (you may experience this a few times a month)
    - o sores inside or on the side of your nose, these are not zits
- *Feet*
    - o painful lumps that you can barely walk
    - o very painful sores on your heel from very dry feet

Symptoms	Morgellons Disease	Fibromyalgia	Lyme Disease	Shingles
Muscle pain, twitching, burning or tightness	X	X	X	
Low pain threshold or tender points	X	X	X	
Pain	X	X	X	X
Draining fatigue Always tired	X	X	X	X
Brain fog Trouble concentrating and remembering	X	X	X	

Symptom				
Worried, feeling nervous or depressed	X	X	X	
Bloating, belly pain, constipation, queasiness, and diarrhea (irritable bowel)	X	X		
Headaches	X	X	X	X
Neck stiffness	X		X	
Runny nose or mucus	X	X		
Dry eyes, mouth, and nose	X	X		
Sensitivity to light, heat, cold, or sound	X	X		X
Peeing more often	X	X		
Numbness or tingling in your face, arms, hands, legs, or feet	X	X	X	X
Joint pain	X		X	
Rash	X		X	X
Sensitivity to light	X		X	X
Fever and chills	X		X	X
Vision issues	X		X	X

(Hernandez, 2019)

Why I Believe Other Diseases Is Morgellons Disease

First things first, every one of these so-called diseases in the medical library I listed, as source unknown how long have these things been on the books without anyone finding what exactly is causing this problem.

I have gone through a lot of information at the medical library and saw many images from many medical websites that makes me wonder how in the world these people could not see the silicon covering their body is alive. This is why *Aspergillus fumigatus* has been running wild and spreading like crazy. Shingles, Lyme disease, fibromyalgia, eczema, dermatitis, and a few others skin diseases are caused by a fungus. I can prove it in a heartbeat. It is unbelievable that these doctors have actually been torturing people for so long. I they doing this for the money or just stupid. Neither choice is good. The only reason I can see this is because I know what I'm looking for. I don't even need to get a specimen out for someone because I had been through it. My health is changing drastically right now. I can't accept BS.

I found a friend who was diagnosed with shingles. I was able to obtain a specimen from that person, which was Morgellons fungi. I had gone to a catered party that had a bald bartender. When I happened to be alone with him in the room, I was able to ask him if could look taken some images from him just for data. I notice that a lot of the bald people have very shiny heads. It always made me wonder if that really was his skin because skin is not supposed to be shiny. That was one of the reasons why I needed to know and I saw exactly what I was looking for.

Think about it this way, you can see a fish being eaten alive by a jellyfish because that jellyfish is transparent. This is why these fungi have been able to hide in plain sight.

AIDS and herpes are also included as one of the diseases that is actually caused by the highly aggressive fungus.

If you have a problem with what I am telling you, prove me wrong. I guarantee that I will still win because I can prove everything I'm saying. This is not my job. I'm doing this because I've spoken to too many people that had been hurt in the medical field. If people have to go through the hell that they're going through you not too far behind because you with a doctor is probably already infected. It's sad that everywhere I go, I have to keep silent even though I could tell people what to do to help themselves.

I was not happy looking at all these ugly images and all the data I gathered just to prove that the world is in trouble and is getting worse. We better get our act together.

Signs You May Be Infected

One of the first sign that you are infected may be itching on the face, around the mouth, crotch, nose, and ankle. You may feel a little itch or something moving around on your behind or back. You start getting gray hairs, but you ignore it because you think you are just getting older. Your sight starts to get worse and need reading glasses. This happened to me years ago when the doctors told me it was just my age, but I now know that it was Morgellons disease. You may feel like things are falling off your body. You may find stuff like dandruff on your clothes (this is not dandruff). You may start finding little cotton balls or lint on your clothes, sweatpants, shirts, and around the house. You may start experiencing stomach problems and bloating. You may experience constipation. This happens because the fungi has clogged your intestines and hardened you stool, which makes it hard for you to go. You may or may not start getting sores that you don't know how you got them.

Just because you don't have visible sores does not mean you don't have them. I have spoken with people that ask if what they were experience was Morgellons disease even though they had no sores. I told them they should start bathing with warm water and baking soda. After these people took their baking soda bath, the hidden sores started showing up. You must understand that you will see sores all the way to the end of the fight. They just keep getting smaller until your body gets rid of them. (Hernandez, 2019)

How Did We Get Here?

For quite some time, scientists and doctors have been misdiagnosing shingles, Lyme disease, dermatitis, eczema, fibromyalgia, AIDS, and many other skin diseases. They also tell you that these things are not contagious. They are dead wrong.

This is why this is now a worldwide pandemic, and I believe that everyone is already infected. Many people start finding long strands of hair around the home and in the car, even if they are bald. Many people are starting to have vision problems, losing hair, and hair turning grayish white. This is not due to old age or genetics. This is an infestation of a fungus.

With the experience that I've had, this has become easy for me to see and identify an infected person. There are many ways I can do this and many ways I can obtain a living sample from anyone within five minutes. I am concerned that if we don't start fighting this now, the world is in danger. This just doesn't affect middle age or older people. It affects everything and everyone, no matter what age, nationality, color, male, or female.

One of the things I've noticed in my studies is that Lyme disease and shingles has been increasing at a very high rate. I know this is happening because they are not treating the source, which is a fungus. How many people have to suffer and die before we start treating the source? If you don't think that people are dying because of these fungi, then why do you think the life expectancy has gone down in the United States in the past three years from drug overdose, suicide, and liver disease? (Hernandez, 2018)

Autoimmune Disorders

Doctors have a habit of jumping to autoimmune disorder every time they cannot explain why your body is not able to fight off whatever is causing your problems. They never thought that maybe your whole body's being overwhelmed by an organism that covers your whole body.

In my conversation with hundreds of people with Lyme disease, shingles, eczema, and a few others diseases, one of the first thing the doctors claim that you may have an autoimmune disorder. This is their go-to answer for everything they don't understand. The doctors are not thinking that your body's immune system is being overwhelmed. Almost like a war, you are outnumbered by a billion to one. You and have no chance of winning, especially when you're fighting something that also has the ability to camouflage itself from your body's natural defense. Like I said before, there is some kind of fungi that are able to masquerade themselves as bacteria, like that scientists from Israel said when he found a fungi that was masquerading as bacteria. This is recorded in the National Library of Medicine.

I hope that my message to the world, the public, and the medical field start using their head and really start treating the people how they should be treated and stop the unnecessary suffering of their patients. Autoimmune deficiency or disorder is not real. What's real is that the body is being overwhelmed by billions of a foreign organism and or bacteria outnumbering your antibodies. Why can't doctors just tell the truth and say, "I don't know what is happening, but I would look into it and see what we can do to help people." (Hernandez, 2019)

Morgellons Disease Treatment and Cure

This process is not going to be an overnight cure. It is going to take a few months, if not two or three years._You are fighting an infestation by a living organism that has your body surrounded inside and out.

One of the biggest problems with the treatment is that there are side effects. One of those effects is the chills. This is something that is going to go all the way through the end. The reason this is happening is because your body is fighting an all-out war with the organism that has stealthy capability to hide from your antibodies. Another one of those effects is that you will feel your body burning. This may happen with your treatment, not because these fungi go through a metamorphosis when it changes into liquid and solid. You may feel weak, very tired, dizzy, and unable to think clearly.

I'm going to list three products I used. I recommend that you start slow because I'm not sure which one cause the problem. I started taking four pills of caprylic acid and undecylenic acid, but I don't recommend this because I was in massive pain for a few hours. The fungus fight back one side of my face was on fire enter solid as a rock. This is why I recommend to start slow. The pain is not good.

- *Undecylenic acid.* Take undecylenic acid three or four times a day. Please start with one pill and work your way up to three or four pills slowly.
- *Caprylic acid.* Take caprylic acid three or four times a day. Start with one pill and work your way up to three or four pills slowly.
- *Monolaurin.* Take monolaurin three or four times a day. Start with one pill and work your way up to three or four pills slowly.
- *Grapefruit seed extract (GSE).* It's up to you on how much to take of grapefruit seed extract, but three or four times a day is recommended.
- *Castor oil.* Rub castor oil on your whole body. Your skin would turn into grains of sand. This treatment will kill the organism.
- *Baking soda bath.* You should put baking soda on your bathwater You can take a bath at least once a day. Soak for about twenty minutes in the tub, gently rubbing your body.
- *Epsom salt bath.* Do the same as with the baking soda.
- *Baking soda and Epsom salt baths.* You can use both baking soda and Epsom salt together, but it would work better than just using one at a time. They both with help to kill the organism.
- *Colloidal silver.* Apply colloidal silver on your eyes and ears to try to force the organism. This organism is hard to kill because your eyes is so sensitive.

This is the treatment that is available to you. You can get this stuff anywhere. You don't need a prescription to fill it. Now this is not going to be a fun time because the organisms is going to fight back. You may experience chills and tiredness after these treatment. You have to understand, you're trying to win war. You're not just trying to kill a little bacteria, you're trying to kill a living organism. This will go on for a long time. There will be a time when it seems that the organism has shrunk enough where it does not affect you. I told a lot of people that they are going to win this battle, they just have to do what I recommended.

There are drugs out there that the doctors could give you but won't because they think you're nuts. They would label what you have as shingles, Lyme disease, eczema, or all other stuff. Morgellons disease is an aspergillosis, caused by an invasive fungi. Once doctors get it through their heads, they will be doing humanity and the world justice. Their job is supposed to help people get well, not send patients to a psychiatrist to tell them they have DOP (delusions of parasitosis).

Here's a list of some of the strongest antifungal drugs that doctors may prescribe to you to treat aspergillosis:

- *Vfend* (generic name, voriconazole). This is what I'm taking right now, which seems to be working very well.
- *Noxafil* (generic name, posaconazole). I also tried this one, but not for a long time.
- *Sporanox* (generic name, itraconazole). I have not tried this.
- *Cresemba* (generic name, isavuconazonium). I had a minor issue with it, but I believe it was because I used the powder version. I started sneezing because the organism was retracting through my sinus. It seemed the organism did not like this drug, which is good.

Why Do I Take These Natural Supplements?

What is caprylic acid?

Caprylic acid comes from coconut and found inside coconut oil. I know a lot of people recommend coconut oil quite a bit. During my research, I discovered that two active ingredients in coconut oil actually affects fungus, one was lauric acid and the other one was caprylic acid. Caprylic acid is one of the most important supplements that you need to kill the fungi. After you take it and gets into your bloodstream, caprylic acid will affect the fungi in two ways: it helps to stop reproduction and also weakens the fungi's cell body wall, killing it.

At the beginning, I had taken both caprylic acid and lauric acid, but soon after, I stopped taking lauric acid because 90 percent is absorbed by your system, only a certain amount turns to monolaurin. For now, just take caprylic acid.

What is undecylenic acid?

Undecylenic acid is made from castor oil and is used widely to treat toenail fungus. Undecylenic acid works just like caprylic acid. It will get into your bloodstream and attack the fungi to stop reproduction and weaken the cell wall.

What is monolaurin?

Monolaurin comes from coconut and mother's milk. Just like undecylenic acid and caprylic acid, it also attacks the fungi by stopping reproduction and rupturing the cell wall of the fungi.

What is GSE?

Grapefruit seed extract is a supplement with a very high antifungal quality. When you take this, you may start seeing things coming out of your body.

When I eat a grapefruit, I even started eating the seeds, which does not taste bad. Grapefruit normally has a little tangy taste, and the grape seed is unexpectedly sweet.

What is colloidal silver?

Colloidal silver was used for quite some time in the past to treat infection. It is made from microscopic silver particles suspended in water.

I invested a lot of money buying colloidal silver because people claimed this was the cure. I spoke with some people I was buying it from and the actual producer. But it was not the cure. It only helped a little to ease the pain. This is why you should use it for your eyes and ears only. It helps to get the fungi out of there.

What is castor oil?

Castor oil was something my mother used to give me when I was a kid. When you rub castor oil on your body, you will start finding grains of salt or even lumps of stuff in your hands and on your body. You want to get that off your body. (Hernandez, 2019)

My Experience and Everything I Tried

When I first started with this, I had a lot of faith in my doctors in treating me and curing whatever I had. That's their job. That's what they went to school for. They will tell you it is just a little rash and give you cream to rub on it. No big deal. I assumed this problem is common. So for years, I went to the doctors to try to get treatment for a rash that kept growing and getting worse. The itch starts driving you nuts, but the doctors gives you another tube of cream that will hopefully take care of it.

This went on for years until I basically stopped working. I was very concerned on how I was going to feed my family and pay my bills. I started panicking, thinking about doing some crazy things because I was concerned I was going to die.

I went to the doctors for many times over until June 2014. That's the time when was I desperate for answers and I realized that these people were not going to help me find it. I was going crazy. I had try to do things to actually get rid of what I knew was a living organism on my body.

I started experimenting with a lot of crazy stuff. Some scared the hell out of me. I thought it was going to die. I poured pure bleach over my head in the shower (please do not try this). I was choking and coughing like crazy. This went on for a little while and scared me. Later on, I drove to the emergency room in the middle the night because I was scared of something moving on my head even though I could not see it. Of course the emergency room staff could not see anything wrong. During this time, I was convinced I had something contagious, even though the doctors said I wasn't. I did not blame the doctors. They just didn't know or couldn't figure it out. My research kept leading me to a few things I originally thought could be an amoeba, parasite, or a fungus, which falls under living organism.

The Mycelium on My Heel

Sometime in 2014, I felt something very painful on the heel of my foot, which made it impossible to walk. The pain was unbearable. I experimented with very warm water in and vinegar as documented in the image below. On the left, you'll see the fungi in a solid form. After soaking in warm water and vinegar, the photo on the right shows the fungus in is liquid mucus form.

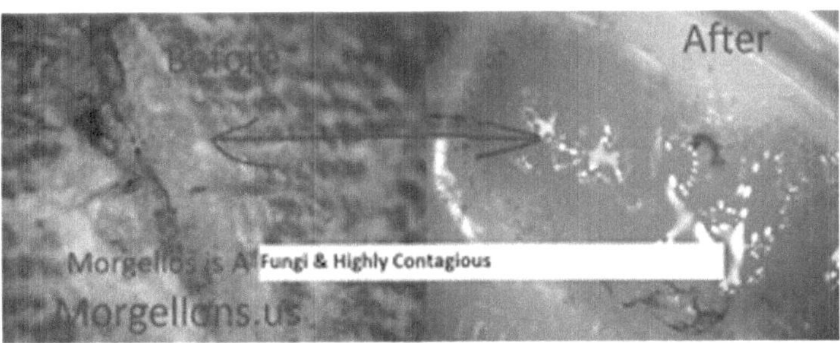

This is one of the reasons why this organism is hiding in plain sight and many people accepting it as normal part of life. Since doctors don't want to accept what is really going on, this is going to get worse before it gets better. At that time, I did not know what I was doing. I did not have the answers I have now. At the end of 2016, I now know that this is a living organism (*Aspergillus fumigatus*) is invading the human body to feed and spread.

The next side-by-side image is of a fungi changing as it is sitting on your skin or what you think that is your skin. This is why your skin feels like silicon. This image was taken sometime in 2013 or 2014. I still didn't know what it was at that time, but we now know that Morgellons disease is caused by a fungus (*Aspergillus fumigatus*).

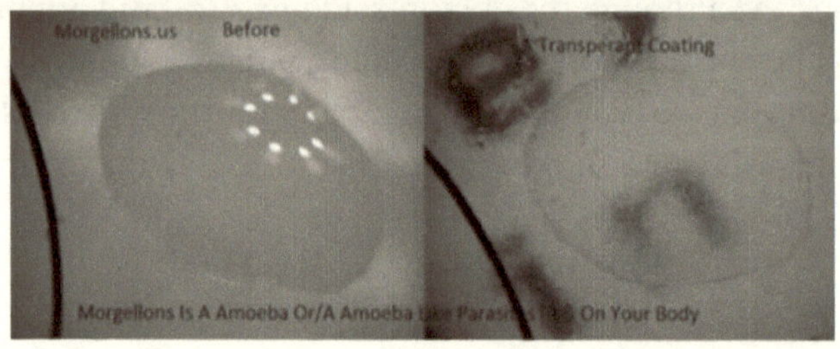

Eczema Is Morgellons Disease

Most kids get eczema nowadays from as early as two months to a few years. It goes away for a short time and comes back during their teenage years. I believe that it has not gone away, just hidden. The problem with this is this thing is in stealth mode. If you look around nowadays, you will find many people suffering from all sorts of the skin problems. You have kids with this cold sores, these little marks in their faces. I ran into a teenager working in Home Depot today. They basically accept this as normal part of life. For someone like myself who spent years researching this stuff, I believe this disease is caused by a fungus living in and on your body. Some medical files claim that eczema or dermatitis is transferred by parents to their infants at childbirth.

Wake up, America. Wake up, world. We need to start working on solving this problem. If we don't vary so people can be very ugly and in regards to it and yes, I mean if you can't see what's going on if the protested a suffering for no reason should not happen.

Look what happened with Joni Mitchell I try to contact them to try to help them to try to open up the rise and what the will was going on with that person. I could not get through to anyone to give them some ideas on what's really going on with her body.

Even on the news, I see guys wearing so much makeup to cover up some of their skin problems. There is a lot of things going on the news. Some people are dying without anyone realizing what's going on. They tell you the symptoms, which are the same with that of Morgellons disease.

You Are Most Likely Already Infected

If you have these symptoms, you are most likely infected:

- hacking cough,
- runny nose or congestion,
- sneezing, like something is in back of your sinus or throat.

The doctors say what you have is an allergy, cold virus, sinus, or the flu. It is not. All these things are from the fungus working its way into your body from the outside. You must start to realize that this is not a cold or flu.

I know, I went through it, and it gets worst. I remember how much money I wasted trying to stop the runny nose and cough with no success. That mucus is a live fungus and spreading quickly. Noticed how many people are walking around you with hacking cough at work, at home—everywhere. You people better wake up.

Diseases That Are Morgellons Disease

These are diseases that has the cause as Morgellons disease (*Aspergillus fumigatus*):

- eczema
- herpes simplex
- dermatitis

- arthritis in joints (including lower back)
- HIV
- shingles
- Lyme disease
- Candida
- *Candida auris*
- AIDS
- canker sores
- cold sores
- blurry vision
- pink eyes.

How to Treat and Kill Morgellons Disease

One of the first things you should do is to bathe at least once a day with baking soda or Epsom salt for about twenty minutes then rub the sores. The sores are really main bodies of the fungi. Fill up the bathroom sink, tub, or a bucket with water, sprinkle baking soda or Epsom salt, pour some on your head, rub it in, and rinse with water. You can pour some over your head and neck too if you have sores in the area. The fungi will just coming off in clumps resembling goo, which you may or may not be able to see in the water.

Most importantly, take the following:

- *Undecylenic acid.* Start slow with 1 capsule and work your way up to 3 or 4 capsules three or to four times a day.
- *Caprylic acid.* Start slow with 1 capsule and work your way up to 3 or 4 capsules three to four times a day.
- *Monolaurin.* Start slow with 1 capsule and work your way up to 3 or 4 capsules three to four times a day.
- *Ground clove or clove oil.* Take once or twice a day with water. Clove is a very potent antifungal.
- *Grapefruit seed extract (GSE).* Take three to four times a day.
- *Colloidal silver.*
- *Castor oil gel pills.*

- Rub *castor oil* on your body and head.
- Rub *clove oil* on your body and head. It may sting so try to keep away from the eyes.

Morgellons the Silent Pandemic

I have spoken to a few hairdressers and asked about people's head and hair. Even though I've never mentioned my findings, one of them started telling me about some guys wanting to get a haircut that had goo coming out of their head. They told me they would come back once it dries. I explained to him that the fungi is basically reproducing at the top of their head. I told him that what they're seeing is actually the multiplication of the mycelium. I shared that I've had that same condition in the past and it was driving me crazy. I had done something that I would not tell the doctor because he made a say this guy is nuts which they already assume that, but I knew my body and I was able to get a hold of one of these sore lips or whatever if you want to call it a sore and what end it up happening when I ripped it open and what came out was a goo, clear liquid that fell of my head. During this time, the person's body may experience chills and even fever, the effects of the body combatting this infection, putting a strain on the body.

While the hairdresser and I were having a conversation, a young person came in to get a haircut. He was close enough got me to get a look at his nose. I noticed that his nose was an ugly looking, but I did not say anything to him about it, just kept talking with the hairdresser until he was done. After the kid was gone, I asked the hairdresser about the kid's nose. He said that the sore on his nose doesn't heal. I continued to ask him if he notice anything wrong with people's heads while he was cutting their hair. He continued his story about the guy who had some liquid coming out of his head. He said that they would wait until the goo dried and turn solid. I finally told him about the highly contagious Morgellons disease. I then suggested that he should always wear gloves no matter who comes in. I told him about the pandemic spreading worldwide easily just by air or contact with any residue. I also asked the hairdresser if he noticed red marks at the back of the neck near the bottom of the head. He admitted that he has noticed the basically a lot of redness in the back of most everyone's neck.

Now look, people, you have to wake up and realize when things are right in front of your face. How much proof do we have to have before we accept the truth that we're in danger of being overwhelmed by a sickness that many people will die from.

In the past, I met someone whose wife was also a hairdresser. He told me that she was concerned because people's head don't look too well. I told him the same thing I told her the hairdresser guy about the pandemic and recommended she should be wearing gloves. Gloves protect the person from getting infected.

I believe that these fungi has already spread worldwide. The only difference is what stage everybody is at.

What to Expect When Treating Morgellons Disease

The cure for Morgellons disease will be a long process. You will see some crazy things happening before and after treatment.

Some people believe that those white flakes falling on their shirt is dandruff. It is not. It is the fungi. Those fuzz balls people find on their clothes or sweatpants are not cotton balls. It is the fungi.

The image below shows one of the hair like threads fiber that comes out of your so call sore which is a the fungi mycelium—main body many people may be able to see this as one of those monsters comes out what you think is your skin, it is not just to ensure you understand what's going on. You will see a shiny coating on your skin. Believe me, it is not your skin. That is the body of the fungi covering your skin with layers of silicon.

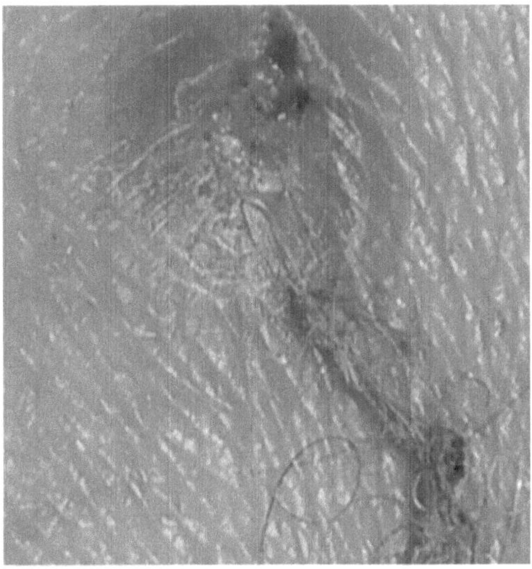

This battle is very scary, especially when you don't know what's going on. This is something that I dealt with every call I had before at the beginning of my battle when it almost had me paralyzed. Some sores you can barely see on your joints. This is the reason why you have major arthritis problems and swelling, all caused by the fungus. If you don't start to treat this before it gets, this will be a living hell and will take you a long time to get rid of.

The medical field has not been treating any of these problems, preferring to diagnose ailments as Lyme disease, shingles, eczema, plaque psoriasis, dermatitis, HIV, herpes, AIDS and many other medical problems. When you go to the government medical library, all of these have been identified as the source. *Aspergillus fumigatus* is the real source of all of these diseases. As I said before, when I went to the doctors to find out what was going on with me, they kept coming up with different scenarios. I could not accept their explanation, even though I'm not a doctor.

Everything I've told you in this book is to help you survive and win the battle of this infestation without losing your mind. Your skin is going to have sores all over your body. Don't panic. You will go through many stages all the way to the end. The fight will take some time, but it won't be that bad once you get to a certain stage when the mass is mainly on top of your head. You won't have the headaches anymore because the main concentration is localized on top of your head and have shrunk substantially.

During the time when I was looking for many ways to kill this fungi, I experimented with many things. In 2014, I tried to share my findings to every pharmaceutical company, but they made is so complicated because they have rules to follow. I could partner with them and get paid to actually do further research, but the problem is that I did not have a degree, nor was I a doctor. At that time, I discovered one of the antifungal treatment that was meant to kill the fungi throughout the body. The company did accommodate me and even got me in touch with one of their specialist from the infectious disease department handling the Ebola epidemic in Africa. I told him one of the effective short-term treatment I found was drinking baking soda. The specialists told me that they lost a lot of people in Africa from overdose of baking soda. I could not remember the exact words.

When I drank baking soda for about a week, it did help me but also weakened my body quite a bit. The fungi was fighting back really hard. Shortly after, I basically emptied everything out. But I also drank a lot of water to ensure I did not get dehydrated. I only took baking soda for a short time because it was draining my body big time, though I felt better. I was always experimenting on different things to cure every ailment I had. There were some crazy things I tried but never told the doctors. I stopped seeing for treatments. I get closer and closer to the answer.

One time, I found a sore on top of my head. Because this thing was driving me crazy, I rip that sore open and a clear goo oozed (please don't do this). This was how I knew about the outer coating on my body. This is one of the reasons people started to look very ugly because this is been spreading slowly right in front of all of us. The world better wake up because soon most of the people would be practically crippled by this monster. This thing doesn't just go after people, it goes after animals, insects, and everything imaginable. What happens if the bees start disappearing, like they already are? This thing may have something to do with it.

I love the eczema commercials. It's great how they can advertise all of the symptoms that most people are being told is all in their head, yet they put an ad that basically makes you look silly because those symptoms are the same things that your doctor tells you exists only in your head. For Lyme disease, they might show you images of a bug (tick). But they don't notice that bug has already been covered by the goo from the fungi... I have read so much data and images of people infected with many diseases, including Lyme disease, shingles, eczema, AIDS, herpes dermatitis, and fibromyalgia. It didn't take long to actually realize that these are all the same; that is, all of them have the same symptoms. It's just named something else. This has to come to an end. Many people are suffering and killing themselves because the doctors are not helping them. We better get our acts together.

I know that many people have all kinds of idea the chemtrail some of them brought it to my attention. But all that stuff did not compute. I could not see anything to tie it to Morgellons disease so I could not say that all that stuff had anything to do with the disease that is infecting you, your home, and everything around you. Just because you don't have it or you don't think you have it, you probably already do. This infestation takes a long time to grow, like the fish being eaten alive by a jellyfish.

When You're Desperate, You Try Anything

I have tried so many crazy things out of desperation. Please do not try them. I bathed with gasoline and turpentine. This really didn't do much for me. Like I said, when you're desperate, you try anything. When something is driving you crazy, you would try anything.

I found out that there are three versions of UV light. UVA and UVB penetrates your skin and is harmful to you. I'm not going to go into details, but they use this in the tanning bed. UVC (warning, you may experience pain in your eyes from the fungi, which could last hours or days) is the one that I experimented with because UVC is used to disinfect and kill bacteria and fungi. I did use it multiple time but don't recommend because it is going to cost your eyes. This is something t you could probably use in your home. UVC kills the fungi by changing its DNA so that it can't replicate itself. Shortly after, flakes came off my skin. The fungus turned white like snow-flakes and fell off my skin. When I extended my arm, flakes fell off. I demonstrated this even at the convention in 2015.

The only reason I did not share some of these things I've tried to anyone is only because I'm trying to protect from hurting people. That's how I came up with the caprylic acid, undecylenic acid, monolaurin, grapefruit seed extract, baking soda, and Epsom salt bath. These things help you kill the fungus on your body.

The People Infected

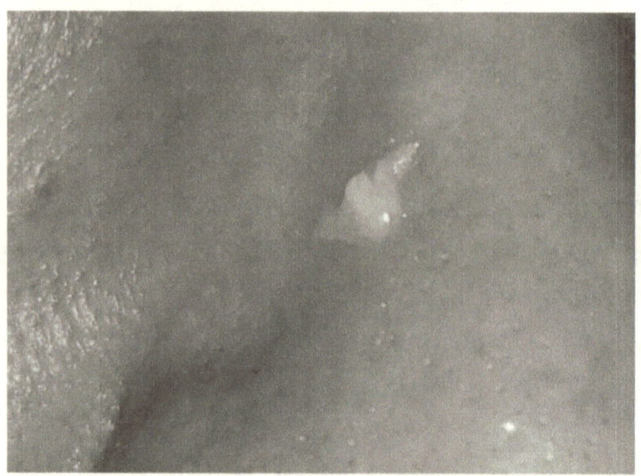

One of the ways to tell whether someone is infected with the fungus is to take a look at their body and head. Bald people are still infected even though you don't see it. Most of these people have a lumpy body. Those lumps are main bodies of the fungi. On a bald head, these lumps would have some dark spots or maybe even sores, which is the fungus. Your head is a little bigger than what it really should be because there is multiple layers that is not part of your body on the head your head is surrounded by a thick layers around the head and multiplied over the years and on the back of the head and neck there might be lumps and red/dark spot this is not just the lump people sometimes you feel something moving on your head and you go to touch it and it scares you so you pull away go back to find it but then it's gone this will happen this does happen.

The last spot you're probably going to kill is the one on top of your head. As you are starting the treatment, you will notice and feel the mass on top of your head shrinking. Once you get to the advanced stage, you will notice your skin feels different throughout your whole body, like it's back to normal. But I recommend you continue with the treatment because this things tend to grow back and will fight you till the end. Keep taking some of like caprylic acid and undecylenic acid because others may still be contagious.

If you haven't notice how ugly people are looking these days, you must not have your eyes open. I see this every day at the store or anywhere I go. I've noticed people who practically have no hair, and women I meet are messed up. If we don't work on this, if we don't get the doctors to take care of people and get rid of this infestation, then we are doomed.

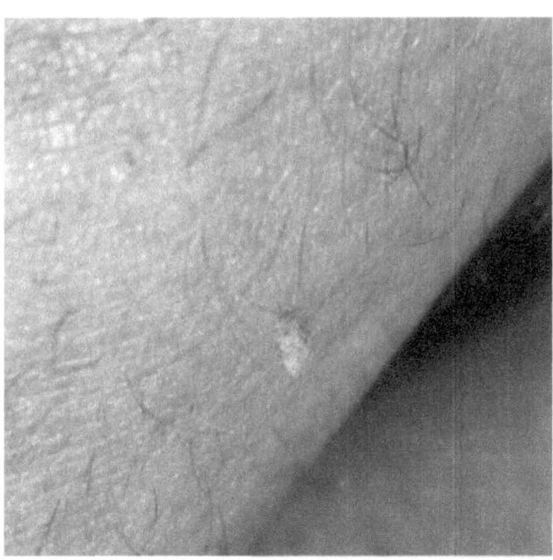

Aspergillus fumigatus is a living organism that has the ability to change at will, from liquid to solid to threads, which makes it complicated for you to understand what's going on. This organism is able to change at will so I wanted to find a known creature that was able to do the same. I found that the sea cucumber was able to change at will from to liquid solid, which gave me something to compare that these fungi is able to do the same.

A Faster Way to Kill It

The doctors are really torturing their patients, whether intentional or not. For the last year and half, I have not been as tortured as a lot of you may be experiencing, but I knew that there was still a mass on my body, mainly on my head. Vfend was still killing the mass but very slowly. Some of that reason was partly my fault because I was still experimenting and trying to find a faster way to kill this monster faster. Even though I'm at the end of the journey, I'm still experimenting on finding the fastest way to kill these fungi without much stress on the person or other living things.

My Final Thoughts and Conclusion on Morgellons Disease

I had found that this fungus is continuously on the prow to find a host to infect. Once a person is infected, the fungi will grow and start spreading everywhere, covering your floors, carpet, chairs—anything it I can get on. What is known about these fungi is nowhere close to how bad the situation is. Morgellons disease, the silent pandemic, has gone unidentified for years in plain sight.

This book is going to tell you everything you need to know how I have eliminated this monster from my body. If I did not start to become my own scientist and doctor in 2014, I would have probably been dead by now. I was losing my mind back then. This infection was making it hard to think due to something called brain fog. My personality changed a lot from the torture, sleeplessness, and the unsightliness of sores on my face and body. The condition made me to hide from family and friends, even though doctors told me that it was not contagious. I knew for a fact that it is that's why I stayed away from everyone because I was concern for my family and friend's health and well-being. Every time I went to a gathering, people kept asking if there is something wrong with me. If I'm okay, I would always say, "Yes, I'm fine."

What I am about to explain to you in this section is going to be my findings off what is growing on everyone's body that the doctors come up with some BS name for. If we do not bring this to light now, life expectancy will continue to decline and the suffering will continue to increase till the end. Most people don't realize they are infected until it has spread far enough to cover the body and multiple layers of your skin, though it is the fungi masquerading as your skin. The mycelium of the fungi forms hairlike threads grow on other parts of the body. The main body of the fungi (mycelium) will grow and move to the top of your head and start max production.

During my experience of trying to figure out what was going on with me, I have done some crazy stuff to end this monster since doctors seem to have their head up their behinds and tell everyone that they are delusional because they don't know what's going on even though they see things that look like open sores on your body. They tell you it's all in your head and not even listen to anything you are saying to them. How the has the medical field fallen so far back? In my early twenties, I remember when they started talking about AIDS and made it very scary to even get involved with anyone as they described it as highly contagious. Now there are things that have been normalized that should have never been.

After years of fighting this crap, I am finally at the end of killing the main body of this organism that has been hidden in plain sight on my body. The big thing is that I have seen that this is not a localized situation. These fungi has infected the human race and all living organism. Most people believe that they got infected when they first start, feeling a lot of the heavy symptoms, which most likely is wrong. At the beginning, you may only start with a minor itch. The infection takes many years to grow. Jock itch, foot fungus, and ringworm are telltale signs that you are infected. It took four or five years for me to exhibit was the first visible symptom. You may start seeing this is when you start getting so-called gray hairs. Your beard is most likely the first place you start seeing it.

This information is going to be hard to take. Most people have gotten accustomed with everything changing in their appearance and accept it as normal, which is not a hundred percent accurate. The information that I'm going to give you will show you that something is wrong. It was hard for me to accept what I was experiencing. It just did not compute. I couldn't accept it as something that I will have to suffer and live with for the rest of my life, not treat or kill it.

Most people don't realize that their body is being coated with a silicon-like living organism. Most people don't notice that their body seems to be growing in size and most of that growth is not yours. During my process, I lost fifty pounds in less than one year. I can't understand how no one notices that their head is getting bigger or that there is a mass growing on their head. Every time I go to the supermarket or basically anywhere, I see these poor people who are losing the hairs, yet no one notices that this a huge mass right on their head.

I always had a couple of lumps throughout my body. I had a couple removed about thirty years ago. My body was covered with a lot of lumps throughout. I used to disregard them because I've always had them. One day I realized that those lumps were not mine, but a fungus growing on my body.

Most people don't realize they have a little something under their nose that that is a living organism living on their body. Scientists or doctors are coming up with BS name and calling that silicon layer covering your body as biofilm. The biofilm is billions of fungal cells covering your body inside and out. The bacteria that these doctors are finding, like Borrelia, is secondary to the source of the fungi, *Aspergillus fumigatus*, which has the ability to change shapes to solid, liquid, threadlike, and siliconlike.

During my quest for answers, I found a sample the fell off for me when I was highly infected. I could not figure out how to get it off the floor, but I wanted it because it was a perfect specimen. They had the different color threads. I surrounded the specimen with plumber's putty but I did not have enough. I added water to get it afloat and separated then I went to Home Depot. When I came back, there was a two-foot hairlike thread that grew from the specimen. It shocked the hell out of me. But this also gave me more answers to the puzzle that I was working on. I wished I could have taken a picture, but when you're in shock, you don't do things you need to do. It was still early during my quest to try to find the answer.

One of those crazy things that I experienced was when I went outside to talk to my neighbor. A bug was flying around me. All the sudden, the fungus grabbed the bug right from my neck and absorbed it. I know my neighbor saw this even though he didn't say anything because I saw the shocked look he had. I know this is crazy, but one moment, there was buzzing and the next, nothing. The bug was gone.

This wasn't really a big shock because some crazy things were happening during my time all high infestation I knew I was right especially when you used to see bugs like ants that will call on your floor which is was a ground-level which meant that I was able to see a lot of bugs that all the sudden would be stuck on the floor I used to wonder what the hell's going on they would not move they would not be able to move this happen a lot of times and I could not understand what was going on this was another clue to my puzzle specially since I started finding a lot of bugs coated in white silicon.

The Cure

How I came up with the cure? Just before I told the doctor to go to hell, I tried everything that they recommended, and it did nothing. After everything they prescribed to me for so many different things, I was able to convince them to give me an antifungal that they cut me off after one prescription because I took a higher dose than they recommended. They had given me Diflucan, which is a good antifungal, but not strong enough. It helped but worked very slowly. During this time, I went nuts, buying everything antifungal medicine I could get my hands on. I started eating a lot of garlic, clove, oregano, turmeric, cumin, cinnamon, and anything I could find that had natural antifungal properties.

How I Treated and Killed This Monster

Like I've said before, I tried a lot of stuff, some that were harsh. I knew that I was fighting a living organism so I tried everything that the doctors prescribed, even though they don't know what they were fighting. Most of the stuff didn't do much. I finally found something that worked. Bathing with vinegar somewhat helped. I was a little scared because I saw white goo on the side of my face near the eye. At the same time, the blue bucket with vinegar and water was effective. Something was coming off my body. That picture of the blue bucket and red cup is proof of the dead fungi. You must understand that your immune system is being overwhelmed and what you're fighting is a living organism surrounding your body billions of them working as one and multiplying even though I was getting a lot of the stuff off my body I would be drain later from my immune system working overtime killing and fighting to rid the foreign organism that invaded my body, you will go through this punishment on all the way through the end till you win.

During this process, I also learned the fungi will work overtime to replicate itself. This monster wasn't just on the outside of my body, it was also inside. I needed to find a way to kill it inside so I drank a lot of apple cider vinegar, which helped but wasn't strong enough. At times I could not sleep because my stomach was hurting. I felt bloated and force myself to throw up, which helped to relieve the pain so I could go back to sleep._When_I looked in the toilet later, I saw was the clear goo that came out of me. I also had a problem with being constipated. This is how I found baking soda, which I drank the next day to force myself to go to the bathroom and get everything out. To avoid getting dehydrated, I always drank a lot of water.

I was able to get in touch with a pharmaceutical company that connected me with a representative who was an expert on Ebola as an infectious disease doctor working in Africa. The doctor told me to be careful with the baking soda because people were dying from drinking a lot of it in Africa. I appreciated the data they have given me. The only reason I could not work with the company was because the hiring process was crazy. The whole pharmaceutical industry is a restricted environment.

I drank baking soda for about a week, which did help, but every time I kill some, the fungi would fight back, trying to regain control of my body. I told people online that they should bathe in baking soda. How much to use is up to you. Submerge as much of your body as you can underwater. The sores are fungi mycelium and you have more than one and a lot of them are hidden. You will win this battle to rid this monster, but you must keep going don't quit you can't have one on your body because it will be replicating again and you will be back in the same scenario again. After you bathe, you should use castor oil all over your body.

You must also take undecylenic acid, which comes from castor oil and a very potent antifungal. Start slow because I took four pills right off the bat and it was not a very fun situation. One part of my face was on fire and in pain. This went on for a while after the first time. The fungi does not like it and will fight back. Undecylenic acid does get into your bloodstream without killing the good bacteria. Caprylic acid is a little weaker than undecylenic acid, but I would recommend to take it slowly too, just in case. Take these three or four times a day. Undecylenic acid is five times stronger than caprylic acid, but is your choice whether you want to take them both or just one. Grapefruit seed extract is another thing that you can take that will help you to force this fungi out of your body. You will start finding things coming out clumps so don't panic if you find these weird silicon things around. Colloidal silver, the stronger the better, will be good for your eyes and ears because the fungi affects your sight. Monolaurin is also another good antifungal that would help to kill these fungi. As time goes on, your sight will probably get better. During this time, you may also see floaters that could be the fungi. Your ears may have things to look like wax but is most likely the fungi.

This is going to be a long battle, but you just can't give up. You will go through hell for little while, but there will be a breaking point where all the sudden when you're getting close to the final stages and get rid of the whole thing from your body. You must remember that you are fighting a living organism that is trying to win. It is an all-out war. You will be experiencing chills and fever off and on all the way through the end. A lot of your pain that you are suffering now will subside, and life may begin to get easier for you.

Now there are multiple antifungal drugs that will help to kill this monster that the doctors could give you. Here is a list of the drugs that I know will help:

- Vfend (generic name, voriconazole)
- Sporanox (generic name, itraconazole)
- Noxafil (generic name, posaconazole)
- Cresemba (generic name, isavuconazonium).

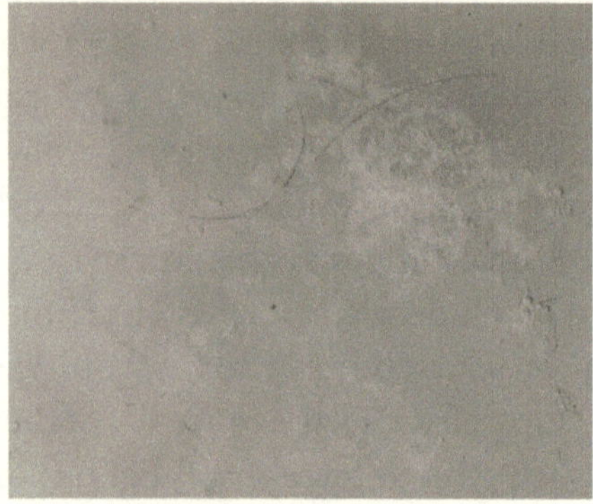

I tried to get the doctors to give me some of these drugs, but they always referred me to psychiatrist. I finally gave up and decided to cure myself. At the beginning, I tried to get voriconazole but it was expensive to get from overseas. I was able to purchase a few pills of Diflucan from Canada but it strained me financially and it was still not strong enough to help kill these fungi quickly. I needed something stronger. There was a new drug call isavuconazonium (Cresemba), a strong antifungal, but it was expensive for me to get it. I was only able to buy a few grams. It cost me a lot to but I had a minor side effect of making me sneeze. I felt the goo coming out of my body. It was not fun. I finally found a way to get 2 kg of flu-conazole (Diflucan) and bought a capsule-making machine to make the pills so I could take them daily. This accelerated my success in killing this monster. They helped a lot, but it was still a slow process. It took ten to twenty years. You are not going to kill this thing over-night until we find some better way to kill this monster.

Most people don't realize that they're infected until it starts to affect your life. This is why the fungi has been spreading like wildfire because it is roaming free and we are not doing anything about it. *Aspergillus fumigates* was number two fungi ten or fifteen years ago, now it is number one. I believe that these fungi are responsible for most diseases throughout the world.

The image above is the fungi when it comes off your body. I know it looks like nothing, but believe me, this is or was a living organism. I've got this off my head, which was the hardest part to kill, with water and baking soda. I just filled the sink with water and baking soda. I didn't really measure how much baking soda I used. I guess I put in about a third of a two-pound baking soda container in the water. Then I used one hand to cup up some water and pour it over my head while rubbing it off as with the other hand. When you are putting your hand in the baking soda water after a mass fell off your head that may scared you, because I had a few times when I found resistance in the water and sometimes run into solid objects for a few seconds and then you look to see what the hell was in the water and you find nothing.

Most people don't even notice that their head, face, and nose is bigger than what is supposed to be. The reason is because you have multiple lawyer a fungi covering the head and body, some of it have grayish hair popping up all over your body. You may start noticing parts of your face turning to goo. The fungi could not maintain its solid form in the baking soda water. It took me fifteen to twenty minutes to do this. I also had mucus that kept coming out of my nose.

Baking soda is the best way to get a lot of these monsters off your body. When I started trying the home remedies, I was not certain I was right about the fungus, even though I had evidence I just needed a confirmation. I got it when I got the DNA result of one of my specimens, which came back in 2016 as the fungus, *Aspergillus fumigatus*. The images below is the fungus *Aspergillus fumigatus* under microscope.

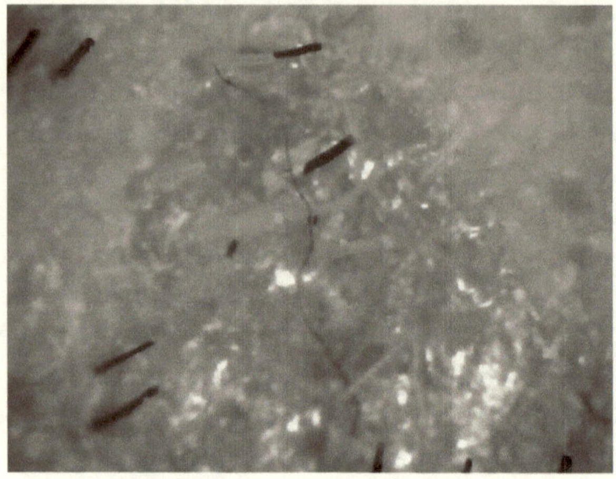

Image above is the mycelium looking like a sore but shiny goo. That is not a pretty sight, some may look even uglier. As you can tell, you can see right through it. The reddish part is your skin while the whitish outer edge is the fungus. This mass on the top your head is able to become solid as a rock and give you huge migraines. I used to experience this a lot.

I spoke with some young lady recently and told her what to do. I warned her she may feel pain, sometimes excruciating pain on other parts of the body. She was in a state of shock because she didn't understand before because she had gone through the same situation as many other people I spoke with. This fungi is a pandemic that is probably killing people that should have no reason to die. If we don't start dealing with this the correct way soon, instead of the BS that the medical field was feeding us and coming up with a different name for the same disease, we are in trouble.

One of the reasons why this was easier for me to figure out what the number of people are infected. This because I never remember people older people getting us ugly as they are now with sores in their heads and everybody going bald.

The image below makes it easier to understand the specimen I had that was crawling up the side of the jar. You could see the metamorphosis from white, semi-solid strand to clear liquid which I call the neural network for each body to be able to communicate.

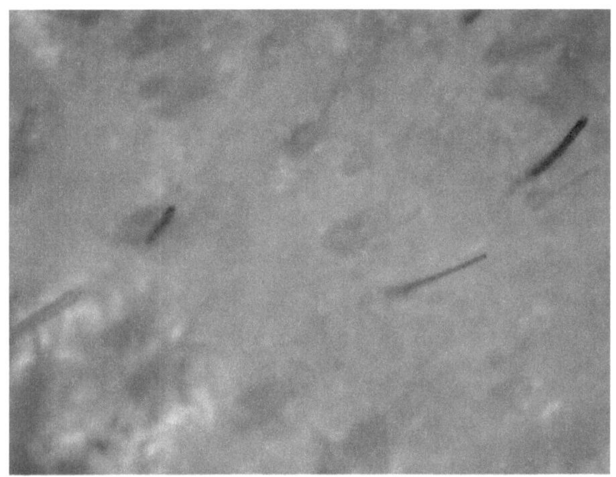

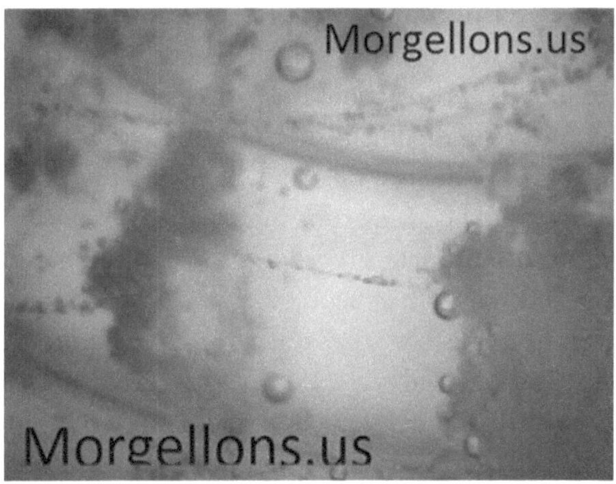

This fungi is spreading in multiple ways: by touch, sexual contact, kissing, or residue left by an infected person. Most people don't even notice that their cell phone has been little particles on it from an infected person, It could appear as little specks white sand on your phone. It is not sand. All you need to do touch it then it attaches itself to you, especially in moist areas. Most of these doctors don't even realize that their patients are already infected. It takes time it will grow and grow.

Morgellons disease is a fungi (*Aspergillus fumigatus*) that can be beaten and get rid, but you must be persistent. It is not going to be an overnight cure. I'm looking into a few more things that I've been experimenting with, but I'm waiting to see if is worth mentioning with what I've shared can defeat this monster. It's just going to take you some time. You must be aggressive and persistent. It is not going to be an overnight success. Even when things drastically change and your life starts getting back to normal, you can't stop because you need to protect yourself from the people that are already infected, which you may not even realize is standing right next to you.

This is sad that we have to become our own healer because the doctors don't understand what's going on. They tell you that your immune is deficient and/or you must be nuts, even though you present them with clear evidence. God help us all. Someone pointed out that I have no other means to corroborate my findings. How am I supposed to get verification when these so-called experts have their head so far up there behind that they can't accept that someone without a degree like them can come up with a solution to some of the most dangerous living organisms in the world?

I guess I must've messed up somewhere because I try to give this information away for free. I spent hundreds of hours, if not thousands, trying to disseminate my findings so I could get help resolve this problem and help other people. Anyone who wants to dispute what I found, don't just say that I'm wrong. I'm more than willing to discuss my findings with you. I don't care if you can have a whole freaking group against me. I will completely prove that I'm right and they're wrong. A lot of people throughout the world will be happy because they can stop the hell that they have been living through and regain a happy life like myself, whose personality has returned.

References

Crum-Cianflone, Nancy, F., MD, MPH. 2009. Clostridium Innocuum Bacteremia in an AIDS Patient. United States National Library of Medicine, National Institutes of Health. https://www.ncbi.nlm.nih.gov/pmc/articles/PMC2732570/

Latgé, Jean-Paul. (1999). Aspergillus fumigatus and Aspergillosis. US National Library of Medicine. https://www.ncbi.nlm.nih.gov/pmc/articles/PMC88920/

About the Author

Armando Hernandez is a very resourceful individual who became infected with something called Morgellons disease.

I am not a doctor. I'm just a guy who does not accept answers and theories that do not compute. I am a United States Navy veteran who was good at what he did I was a troubleshooter.

In the late 1800s, a man discovered a cure for rabies and saved a young boy who was bitten by a rabid animal. Because the man was not a doctor, they tried to throw him in jail, even though he saved the kid's life and created the vaccine for rabies.

I am running into the same issue. Just because I'm not a doctor, I seem to have no right to know what is happening to my own body. What I found is accurate and indisputable evidence that will help millions of people suffering and living in hell just because the doctors and scientists close their eyes on something that is obvious.

Like I said, I'm not a doctor. I'm not stupid enough to be led to jump off a cliff by someone else just because they have a degree. My findings is not a theory; it is fact, and it will be proven so in the near future.